Simulation in Robotic Surgery

a comparative review of simulators of
the da Vinci surgical robot

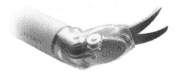

**ROGER SMITH, PhD &
MIREILLE TRUONG, MD**

Modelbenders Press

Modelbenders Press books may be purchased for business and promotional use or for special sales. For information please contact the publisher.

Visit our web site at **www.modelbenders.com**

Cover and interior designed by Adina Cucicov at Flamingo Designs

da Vinci Skills Simulator photos ©2013 Intuitive Surgical, Inc. Used with permission.

dV-Trainer Simulator photos ©2013 Mimic Technologies, Inc. Used with permission.

RoSS Simulator photos ©2013 Simulated Surgical Systems, LLC. Used with permission.

The Library of Congress has cataloged the paperback edition as follows:

Smith, Roger & Truong, Mireille
    Simulation in Robotic Surgery.
    1. Simulation 2. Robotic Surgery 3. Medical Technology
    4. Medical Education
    I. Roger Smith II. Title

ISBN: 978-1-938590-03-0

Acknowledgements

The authors want to thank the following representatives of each simulator company for their assistance in collecting data, images, and videos, as well as verifying the accuracy of the contents of the book. Peter Dominick, Intuitive Surgical Inc.; Jeff Berkley, Mimic Technologies, Inc.; and Kesh Kesavadas, Simulated Surgical Systems, LLC.

Table of Contents

Introduction

For every complex and expensive system, there emerges a need for training devices and scenarios that will assist new learners in mastering the use of the device and understanding how to apply it with value. This has proven to be true in aviation, nuclear power control, and medicine among other fields. Laparoscopic surgery simulators have played a valuable role in improving the practice of surgery over the last 20 years and the same trends and values will likely apply in robotic surgery. The complexity, criticality, and cost associated with the effective application of the da Vinci surgical robot have stimulated the commercial creation of simulators which replicate the operations of this robot. Each of these simulators provides a slightly different perspective and solution to the problem.

This book explores the characteristics and differences between all of the currently available devices. The details provided here are structured to equip readers with sufficient knowledge about the simulators to make their own decisions about which best meets their needs. Each of them possesses unique traits which make them valuable solutions for different types of users. It is not our intent to make a universal recommendation of one device over the others. Readers should draw their own conclusions based on their unique needs for a device.

The three current simulation devices for the da Vinci robot are the:

- da Vinci Skills Simulator (Intuitive Surgical Inc.),
- dV-Trainer (Mimic Technologies Inc.) and
- Robotic Surgery Simulator (Simulated Surgical Systems LLC).

These are commonly referred to as the DVSS or "Backpack", dV-Trainer, and RoSS respectively (Figure 1).

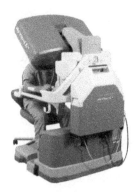 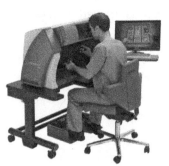 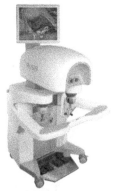

| DVSS, Intuitive Surgical Inc. | dV-Trainer, Mimic Technologies Inc. | RoSS, Simulated Surgical Systems LLC |

Figure 1. Simulators of the da Vinci surgical robot

Each of these devices is manufactured by a different company and provides a unique hardware and software solution for training and surgical rehearsal. The capabilities and features of each are described in this book and summarized in Table 1.

Table 1. Simulator Feature Comparison

	DVSS	dV-Trainer	RoSS
System Manufacturer	Intuitive Surgical Inc.	Mimic Technologies Inc.	Simulated Surgical Systems Inc.
Specifications (Simulator only)	Depth 7" Height 25" Width 23" 120 or 240V power	Depth 36" Height 26" Width 44" 120 or 240V power	Depth 44" Height 77" Width 45" 120 or 240V power
Specifications (Complete System as shown in Figure 1)	Depth 41" Height 65" Width 40" 120 or 240V power	Depth 36" Height 59" Width 54" 120 or 240V power	Depth 44" Height 77" Width 45" 120 or 240V power
Visual Resolution	VGA 640 x 480	VGA 640 x 480	VGA 640 x 480
Components	Customized computer attached to da Vinci surgical console	Standard computer, visual system with hand controls, foot pedals.	Single integrated custom simulation device
Support Equipment	da Vinci surgical console, custom data cable	Adjustable table, touch screen monitor, keyboard, mouse, protective cover, custom shipping container	USB adapter, keyboard, mouse
Exercises	35 simulation exercises	51 simulation exercises	52 simulation exercises.
Optional Software	PC-based Simulation management	Mshare curriculum sharing web site	Video and Haptics-based Procedure Exercises (HoST)

	DVSS	dV-Trainer	RoSS
Scoring Method	Scaled 0-100% with passing thresholds in multiple skill areas	Proficiency-based point system with passing thresholds in multiple skill areas	Point system with passing thresholds in multiple skill areas
Student Data Management	Custom control application for external PC. Export via USB memory stick.	Export student data to delimited data file.	Export student data to delimited data file.
Curriculum Customization	None	Select any combination of exercises. Set passing thresholds and conditions.	Select specifically grouped exercises. Set passing thresholds.
Administrator Functions	Create student accounts on external PC. Import via USB memory stick.	Create student accounts. Customize curriculum.	Create student accounts. Customize curriculum.
System Setup	None.	Calibrate controls.	Calibrate controls.
System Security	Student account ID and password.	PC password, Administrator password, Student account ID and password.	PC password, Administrator password, Student account ID and password.
Simulator Base Price	$85,000	$95,000	$107,000
Support Equipment Price	$502,000	$9,100	$0
Total Functional Price	$587,000	$104,100	$107,000

[Note: Data is for systems available as of April 2013.]

Section 1:
System Design

Da Vinci Skills Simulator (Intuitive Surgical Inc.)

The da Vinci Skills Simulator (DVSS) consists of a customized computer package that attaches to the back of the surgeon's console of an actual da Vinci Si robot. This simulator connects to the surgeon's console via a single proprietary networking cable identical to that used to connect the components of the actual robotic surgical system.

Advantages
Attached simulators of this type are usually referred to as "embedded trainers" because they take advantage of the equipment that has already been constructed, purchased, and installed for the operation of the real system. These kinds of simulators are especially common in military facilities which face limited space and weight constraints. They can significantly reduce the hardware that must be purchased solely for simulation purposes. The U.S. Navy uses these kinds of simulators aboard ships to reduce weight and space requirements, enabling them to train while the ship is at sea.

Another significant advantage of an attached simulator is that it allows the trainee to use the actual controls from the real system to control the simulation. This insures that the training experience is almost identical in feel to the real system, which can contribute to higher transfer of skills from the training sessions to the use of the real system. In learning to use the simulator system, the trainee also has a minimum amount of unique information to learn about the training device. A larger degree of the simulator experience actually contributes to proficiency with the real system.

Finally, there is a cost advantage for the simulator device itself. Because much of the hardware and software expenses are already embedded in the real system, the simulator can be very economical to purchase.

Disadvantages

Attached simulators like the DVSS also come with inherent disadvantages to balance their positive traits.

The largest drawback is the availability of a real system to be able to use the simulator. An attached DVSS simulator cannot be used without access to a real surgeon's console. da Vinci robots are expensive devices which hospitals typically attempt to maximize use of in order to recoup their investment. In a very active surgical hospital, it can be difficult to obtain access to a surgeon's console to support training with this simulator.

The DVSS is designed to connect to the surgeon's console using the same proprietary networking cable that connects the major robot components. This makes the attachment and set-up process very easy for clinicians to master. However, it also means that the DVSS can only be used with the Si model surgeon's console. The previous S and Standard models use a different set of cables which are not compatible with the simulator.

Similar to the military's experience with embedded and attached simulators, heavy usage of the DVSS comes with a corresponding heavy use of the surgeon's console. The Army and Navy have discovered that these types of simulators put more usage hours on real equipment controls which lead to more maintenance costs for those devices. Since it is possible to train almost constantly, the real equipment experiences usage rates that can be many times higher than normal for the equipment. Because the da Vinci systems operate under a maintenance contract that covers all services, the additional costs of maintenance are not born by the hospital owner, but by the equipment vendor. The primary impact to the owner would only be in the area of availability for both real surgeries and training events due to downtime associated with maintenance.

As mentioned under advantages, the cost of an attached simulator is typically much lower than other forms. But that is countered by the fact that the customer must purchase or have available a real piece of equipment to support the use of the simulation.

dV-Trainer (Mimic Technologies Inc.)

The dV-Trainer is a separate, stand-alone simulator of the da Vinci robot. The surgeon's console, controls, and vision cart are mimicked in hardware, while a 3D software model replicates the functions of the robotic arms and the surgical space.

Mimic developed the initial simulator software for the DVSS and used the same package in version 1.0 of their own dV-Trainer. As a result, the exercises in those versions of the systems are nearly identical. The current version 2.0 of the dV-Trainer has a number of new exercises which are not found in the DVSS and the graphics have been upgraded so the visual presentation is no longer identical. The differences in visual presentation can be seen in the figures later in the book.

The dV-Trainer consists of three major pieces of equipment and a number of smaller support pieces. The largest pieces are the "Phantom" hood which replicates the vision and hand controls of the da Vinci surgeon's console, the foot pedals of the surgeon's console, and a high-performance desktop computer which generates the 3D images and calculates the interactions with the surgeon's controls. Smaller support equipment includes a touch screen monitor, keyboard, and mouse to enable an instructor to guide the student through exercises and allow an administrator to manage the data that is collected. There are also a network router and video splitter that connect all of the equipment together. Finally, there is an optional adjustable table with a mount for the PC, monitor, networking equipment, and the Phantom head. This adjustable table is offered as an option for the simulator, but it provides advantages which make it a very advantageous option. This table allows ergonomic adjustments which closely replicate those of the real robot. The table also makes the entire system much easier to package, move within a facility, or ship to other sites.

Because the dV-Trainer replicates both the hardware and software of the da Vinci robot, it is a much larger system than the DVSS alone, though smaller than a real surgeon's console with the DVSS attached. It has the advantage of providing a training system that is completely independent of the need for any piece of the real surgical robot. The simulator can be configured to imitate either the S or the Si model of the da Vinci robot.

The disadvantage of this kind of system is that all simulated hardware is not quite the same as the real equipment. There is always a trade-off between the lower price and the perfect accuracy of a simulator. Also, the simulator must be updated separately when the real equipment is modified.

A user or student can perform most of the exercises on the dV-Trainer that are available on the DVSS, along with many newer exercises that are not available on the DVSS. Both simulators offer new suturing exercises, though they are different for each simulator.

Robotic Surgical System (Simulated Surgical Systems LLC)

The RoSS is also a complete, stand-alone simulator of the da Vinci robot. This device is designed as a single piece of hardware that has a similar design to the surgeon's console of the robot. The hardware device includes a single 3D computer monitor, hand controls that are modified commercial force feedback devices, pedals that replicate either the S or the Si model of the da Vinci robot, and an external monitor for the instructor. Customers must purchase either the S or Si version of the device.

The company has developed a set of 3D virtual exercises that are unique from those found in both of the other simulators. They also provide an optional video-based surgical exercise in which the user is guided through the movements necessary to complete an actual surgical procedure. At this writing, these modules are available for radical prostatectomy, cystectomy, and hysterectomy. These guided videos take advantage of the force feedback capabilities of the hand controllers to push and pull the student's hands to follow the simulated instruments on the screen. They require the student to perform specific movements accurately during the video before the operation will proceed.

Section 2:
Simulation Exercise Modules

Each simulator allows an administrator or instructor to manage and organize student performance according to unique login credentials for the student. Alternatively, they all have a universal "guest" account to make the system accessible to anyone, but without the ability to uniquely identify and track the performance of a specific student.

Once logged into each system, the instructor or the student navigates the instructional materials using the menu systems illustrated in Figure 2. Since the Intuitive Skills Simulator (DVSS) and the Mimic dV-Trainer provide very similar exercises and organizations, the navigation through the exercises is similar in form, though different in visual appearance. The RoSS simulator uses a very unique arced orbital menu for progressing through exercises.

Each simulator provides on-system instructions for every exercise in the form of textual documents and video demonstrations with spoken audible instructions.

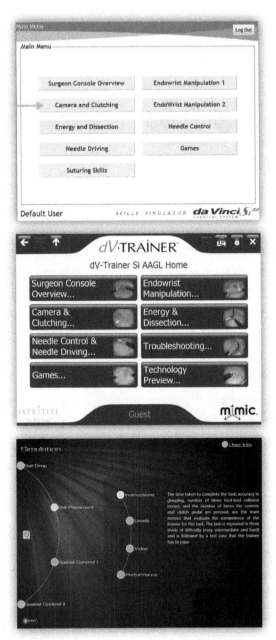

Figure 2. Comparative Simulator Exercise Menus (DVSS, dV-Trainer, RoSS)

DVSS

The DVSS contains 35 exercises organized into nine categories. These begin with introductory video and audio instructions on how to use the robotic equipment, and move through progressively more difficult skills.

Table 2. DVSS Exercise Categories

Surgeon Console Overview	An introduction to the controls of the da Vinci robot.
Endowrist Manipulation 1	Basic hand movements and usage of the wristed instruments.
Camera and Clutching	Basic foot clutching for both the camera and the third arm.
Endowrist Manipulation 2	Intermediate use of the hands and wristed instruments.
Energy and Dissection	Use of the energy pedals and associated instruments.
Needle Control	Focused exercises for dexterous manipulation of a curved surgical needle.
Needle Driving	Repetitive exercises for needle driving.
Games	Challenging and entertaining game environments to apply the skills learned.
Suturing Skills	Suturing exercises with needle, following suture, knot-tying, and tissue closure.

To prepare the student for success in each exercise, the simulator offers written instructions on the objective of each exercise prior to performance. There is also a narrated video of an instructor performing the exercise while explaining the necessary steps.

Upon completion of each exercise, the system automatically proceeds to a scoreboard showing the student's performance on the exercise. Details on the scoring systems of each simulator are discussed later in the book.

Figure 3 presents screenshots of some of the key exercises in the simulator. These include the Ringboard, Ring Walk, Energy Dissection, and Interrupted Suturing exercises. The suturing exercises on this simulator are a new addition which was developed by Simbionix USA Inc. for integration into the DVSS. This expansion of the system was also meant to demonstrate the ability of the hardware platform and underlying management software to blend together simulation exercises and scoring systems created by different vendors.

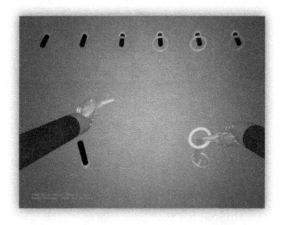

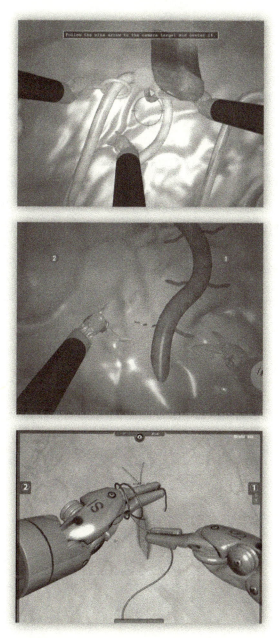

Figure 3. Selected DVSS Exercise Images

dV-Trainer

Most of the simulation software for Intuitive's DVSS was developed by Mimic Technologies. Therefore, version 1 of the DVSS and the dV-Trainer contained nearly identical exercises, closely matching menu systems, and identical scoring mechanisms. However, over time the two sets of software have diverged and the current versions of the simulators differ in functionality and appearance. The current version of the dV-Trainer (v 2.0) contains 51 exercises organized into nine categories. This device also includes video and audio instructions on how to use the robotic equipment, moving through progressively more difficult skills.

Table 3. dV-Trainer Exercise Categories

Surgeon Console Overview	An introduction to the controls of the da Vinci robot.
Endowrist Manipulation	Basic and intermediate use of the hand controllers and wristed instruments.
Camera and Clutching	Basic foot clutching for both the camera and the third arm.
Energy and Dissection	Use of the energy pedals and associated instruments.
Needle Control	Focused exercises for dexterous manipulation of a curved surgical needle.
Needle Driving	Repetitive exercises for needle driving.
Troubleshooting	Introduction to error recovery on the da Vinci robot.
Games	Challenging and entertaining game environments to apply the skills learned.
Suturing Skills	Suturing exercises with needle, following suture, knot-tying, and tissue closure.

Just as with the DVSS, the dV-Trainer simulator offers written instructions on the objective of each exercise prior to performance. There is also a narrated video of an instructor performing the exercise while explaining the necessary steps. Upon completion of each exercise, the system automatically proceeds to a scoreboard showing the student's performance on the exercise.

Figure 4 presents screenshots of some of the key exercises in the dV-Trainer simulator. These include the Ringboard, Matchboard, Tubal Anastomosis, and Energy Switching exercises.

Though many of the exercises are identical between the DVSS and the dV-Trainer, the graphics resolution and details have been improved in version 2.0 of the dV-Trainer software. Since this system is driven by a commercial PC which can be upgraded rather easily, it is possible for the software to evolve and be replaced more easily than for a custom hardware package like the DVSS which would require upgrades to some of the components inside the customized device.

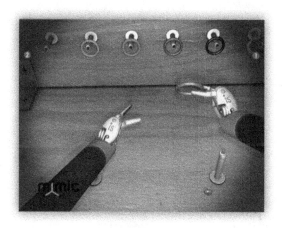

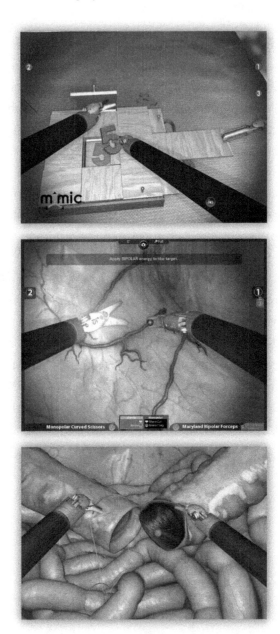

Figure 4. Selected dV-Trainer Exercise Images

RoSS

The RoSS simulator contains 52 unique exercises, organized into 5 categories, and arranged from introductory to more advanced, just as in the other two simulators. The RoSS system of exercises is unique in that they list fewer named exercises, but provide three different levels for most of them. Each of these levels is actually a variation on the exercise design in which Level 1 is the easiest, Level 2 is intermediate, and Level 3 is advanced.

Table 4. RoSS Exercise Categories

Orientation Module	Introduction to the surgeon controls of the da Vinci robot.
Motor Skills	Development of precise controls of the instruments, including spatial awareness.
Basic Surgical Skills	Instruction on handling a needle, using electrocautery pedals and instruments, and the use of scissors on the robot.
Intermediate Surgical Skills	Control of the fourth arm, blunt tissue dissection, and vessel dissection.
Hands-on Surgical Training	Video and haptic-guided instruction through specific surgical procedures.

Similar to the other simulators, the RoSS includes a narrated video showing an instructor performing the exercise. Upon completion of an exercise, the simulator automatically proceeds to the scoreboard for the exercise.

The RoSS contains a unique capability that is not found in either of the other simulators. The company refers to this as "Hands-on Surgical Training" or "HoST." This is an integration of surgical skills exercises with a video of an actual surgery. The company offers a HoST module showing radical prostatectomy, cystotomy, and radical hysterectomy. Videos of actual surgical procedures play in the surgeon's visual space. These are overlaid with animated icons which instruct the student to perform specific actions during the progression of the surgery video. The necessary actions are prompted with audio instructions. For the HoST exercise to progress, the student must perform the specific actions at specific times. The simulator will pause the video and allow the student to repeat the action until it is performed as required by the instructions.

The hand controllers of the RoSS simulator are created by modifying a commercially available 3D haptic computer input device called the Omni Phantom™. This product uses internal motors and gears to apply haptic feedback to the hand movements of the user. For the HoST exercises, the simulator uses this capability to move the student's hands in synch with the movements of the surgeon's instruments in the master video.

Figure 5 provides screenshots of the Motor Skills Ball Placement, Intermediate Vessel Dissection, 4th Arm Tissue Retraction, and HoST Radical Prostectectomy.

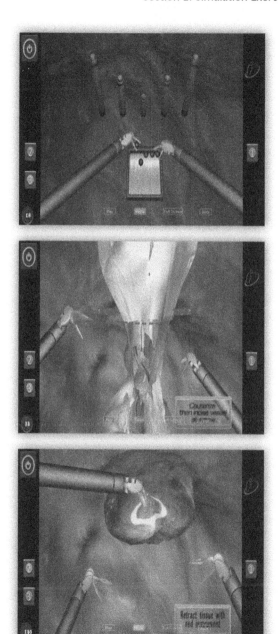

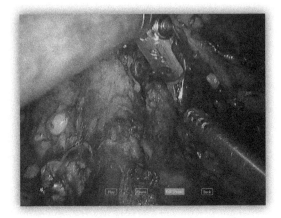

Figure 5. Selected RoSS Exercise Images

Section 3:
Proficiency Scoring

E ach of the three simulators provides a different scoring method. All three use the host computer to collect data on the performance of the student at the controls in multiple performance areas. With this data, they provide a score for specific performance traits, as well as combining all of these into a single composite score of performance for the entire exercise. The algorithm used to create this composite score is described in the user's manuals of each of the simulators. Examples of each of these scoreboards are shown in Figure 6.

Within a simulator, many of the scoring metrics are applied to every exercise, such as the time to complete the exercise. But some exercises have unique metrics that are not applicable to all of the other exercises, such as blood loss volume. In this book we will describe some of the more universally applied metrics, though not all of the unique measurements which are collected for every exercise. Interested readers can consult the simulator's manual for detailed descriptions of all of the metrics across all of the exercises.

In addition to the objective metrics that can be collected by the computer, the developers of each simulator have been challenged to provide thresholds which indicate whether the student's score is considered a "passing" or "failing" performance. All three have identified threshold scores which would indicate acceptable and warning scoring levels. These are commonly interpreted as "passing" (above acceptable threshold) and "failing" (below warning threshold), with a "warning" area between the two thresholds. These thresholds create green, yellow, and red performance areas which can be used to visually communicate the quality of the student's performance in each area of measurement. Each simulator also provides a single composite score for the entire exercise.

For most exercises on all three simulators, higher measurements of performance, such as the time to complete, instrument travel distance, and blood loss, indicate poorer performance; while lower values in these areas indicate better performance. As a result, the collected metric needs to be reversed to create a point system which gives high points for good performance and low points for poor performance. The method used to achieve this is described in the simulator's user manual for the dV-Trainer and can be solicited from the manufacturer for the other two systems.

Each of the simulators gives the student a single overall score for performance on an exercise. To achieve this, an algorithm was needed to combine very different types of metrics. For example, the number of seconds to complete an exercise needs to be combined with liters of blood loss, centimeters of instrument movement, number of instrument collisions, and other similarly varied metrics. As in most educational environments, this is achieved by converting each metric into a score which falls between some defined minimum and maximum value. Most people understand this concept from their academic experience in which all assignments were graded in the range from 0% to 100% or between 0 points and the maximum total points for all assignments. These normalizations make it possible to create a single composite score of the student's performance across multiple assignments. This same approach has been used in the simulators, where the resulting composite metric may be a total point score or a percentage.

The simulator manufacturers all work with experienced robotic surgeons to assist in establishing the relative values of each measure used in the composite score, just as they did for the threshold levels described earlier. Because these evaluations are the opinions of the specific people who have collaborated with the company on the development of the system, the dV-Trainer and the RoSS both provide the ability for a system administrator to adjust these levels to meet the needs of unique curriculum, courses, and students being evaluated.

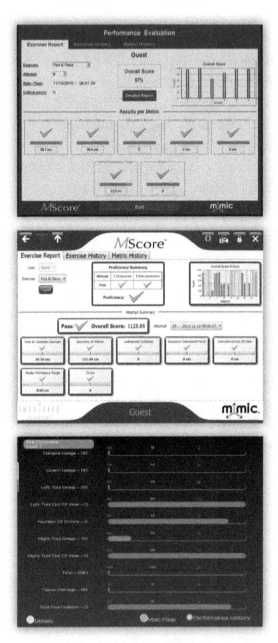

Figure 6. Comparative Simulator Scoreboards (DVSS, dV-Trainer, RoSS)

DVSS

As described earlier, the DVSS performance scoring method has a number of metrics which are applied to every exercise and others which are only used for exercises in which they are relevant. Table 5 presents the metrics which are available on all exercises. For details on the more specialized metrics, the reader should consult the user's manual for this simulator.

Table 5. DVSS and dV-Trainer Scoring Method

Overall Score	Composite evaluation of the exercise performance.
Time to Complete Exercise	Number of seconds to complete the exercise.
Economy of Motion	Number of centimeters of instrument tip movement.
Instrument Collisions	Number of times that the instruments touched each other.
Excessive Instrument Force	Number of seconds that excessive robotic force was applied against objects in the environment.
Instrument Out of View	Number of centimeters that an instrument tip moved outside of the viewing area.
Master Workspace Range	Radius in centimeters than contains the movement of the instrument tips.
Drops	Number of objects dropped from the grasp of the instruments.

Because the DVSS is a closed, turn-key system with an ease of use similar to the actual surgical robot, most of the data displays and threshold adjustments found in the other simulators are not available in this device. Generally, the simulator settings are determined by the manufacturer and cannot be changed by the user.

dV-Trainer

Originally, the DVSS and the dV-Trainer shared the same scoring method, but more recent versions of the dV-Trainer offer both this original "version 1" scoring method, as well as a new "version 2" method based on the proficiency measured from experienced surgeons. The skills measured are the same, but the interpretation of those into a score is different. The instructor can select the preferred scoring method for each curriculum that is constructed in the dV-Trainer.

Users will notice that the newer scoring method uses total points earned rather than percentages. The passing and warning thresholds can be adjusted by the administrator. The philosophy, validity, and effects associated with these settings are more detailed than is necessary for understanding the use of the simulator. Interested readers should consult the user's manual and published literature for details on the two scoring mechanisms.

RoSS

The principles behind the scoring system on the RoSS are the same as those for the DVSS and the dV-Trainer. However, most of the metrics collected are different. The standard measurements are shown in Table 6. Like each of the other simulators, there are multiple displays of the performance data for a student. The initial display presented at the completion of an exercise shows a horizontal bar which is colored green, yellow, or red to indicate passing or failing. The magnitude of the bar is a rough measure of the quality of performance. Additional displays show the numeric score and its relative position to a passing threshold.

Table 6. RoSS Scoring Method

Overall Score	Composite evaluation of the exercise performance.
Camera Usage	Optimal movement of camera.
Left Tool Grasp	Optimal number of tool grasps with left hand tool.
Left Tool Out of View	Distance left hand tool is out of view.
Number of Errors	Number of collision or drop errors in an exercise.
Right Tool Grasp	Optimal number of tool grasps with right hand tool.
Right Tool Out of View	Distance right hand tool is out of view.
Time	Time to complete the exercise.
Tissue Damage	Number of times that instruments damaged tissue with excessive force or unnecessary touches.
Tool-Tool Collision	Number of times tools touched each other.

As with the other two simulators, special metrics are used when they are relevant to a specific exercise. These are not described here, but interested readers can solicit these from the manufacturer.

Section 4:
Simulator System Administration

All of the simulators contain system configuration and student management functions which require a special administrator account to access and modify. These allow instructors to create curriculum and scoring methods which are unique to the lessons they are offering. They also allow an instructor or administrator to create new student accounts and export student scores for evaluation and analysis outside of the simulator device. Some course instructors use this capability to create custom performance reports for students who attend the courses.

DVSS

For the DVSS, most of the administrator functionality is fixed within the delivered system. The administrator can create specific user profiles for the simulator using a dedicated program on a separate external PC. This program, the "da Vinci Skills Simulator Manger", allows the administrator to create a profile for the user. The profile can then be loaded onto a USB memory stick and inserted into the USB port on the DVSS. The simulator will automatically read this data in and display the user names at the login screen.

Similarly, the USB memory stick can be inserted into the DVSS and the performance data collected from exercises performed by each user will be automatically loaded onto the USB stick. This stick can then be inserted in the PC and the data will be loaded into the management software on the external PC and exported to a delimited file for formatting and analysis in a spreadsheet program.

The entire transfer process is automated such that the contents of the USB stick are completely erased and reloaded each time it is inserted into the PC or the DVSS. The stick cannot safely be used for any purpose other than as the transfer mechanism between the two devices. This method is meant to create an ease of use similar to the real robot.

dV-Trainer

The administrator on a dV-Trainer has the ability to create new user accounts, specify S or Si representation, create new curriculum, set passing thresholds, and export user data for analysis.

The simulator contains 51 exercises, any combination of which can be organized into a curriculum for a specific course. The administrator creates the new curriculum name and then adds each exercise that should be part of the curriculum. This set of exercises can be organized into phases or folders to match the course that is being taught. For example, an instructor may have a curriculum that consists of a warm-up with easy exercises, pre-course evaluations, and post-course evaluations. These would appear as three separate sections within the curriculum.

The administrator can export data from the simulator according to multiple criteria. The export may include all of the data on the machine, or subsets defined by the unique user ID, date range, completion status, or a specific exercise.

The capabilities provided for an administrator of the dV-Trainer are significantly more robust than those available on the other two simulators.

RoSS

The RoSS administrator account is used to create student accounts. Each user can then be assigned a specific subset of the entire simulator curriculum.

For the RoSS system, the administrator can assign portions of the curriculum hierarchy which are applicable to a specific user. The curriculum is organized such that customization consists of selective subsets of the hierarchy of exercises, rather than the ability to select specific exercises in unique combinations.

The administrator can also edit the passing thresholds for each exercise. This allows a site to create curriculum which is considered passing for practitioners at different levels, such as medical students, residents, attendings, and specialists.

The scores can be exported as individual delimited data files for each student account. These can then be removed from the system for analysis and recording.

Section 5:
Validation of Devices

Virtual reality simulators have been shown to be effective tools for training in multiple fields such as aviation and the military. These have been used for new skills acquisition as well as maintenance of skills in a risk-free learning environment. The surgical field has recently shown the value for simulation, most notably demonstrated for laparoscopic training. Several studies have demonstrated the benefits of virtual reality surgical simulators such as shorter operating times, decreased learning curve, and fewer medical errors. With the advancement of surgical robotic technology and its rapid implementation as a surgical tool, comes the need for adequate and effective training in order to ensure patient safety. It would follow that the benefits shown for laparoscopic surgical simulation would parallel those for robotic surgical simulation. Recent research demonstrates that robotic simulators are valid training tools and suggests that robotic surgical simulation can help bridge the gap between the safe acquisition of surgical skills and effective performance during live robot-assisted surgery.

Validation studies serve to determine whether a simulator can actually teach or assess what it is intended to teach or assess. There are generally accepted validity classifications, which include face, content, construct, concurrent and predictive validity (McDougall, 2007). Face and content validity are considered subjective approaches while the other three are objective approaches to validation. Face validity evaluates the simulator's realism via informal assessment by non-experts. Content validity evaluates the simulator's appropriateness as a teaching tool via formal assessment by experts. Concurrent validity determines the degree to which the simulator correlates to the "gold standard" as an assessment tool while predictive validity determines the degree to which the simulator correlates to future performance of transferable skills to the operating room. Finally, the most valuable validation approach is construct validity, which is defined as the ability for the simulator to discriminate between various levels of experience, i.e. novice, intermediate, and expert.

Table 7 provides a summary of the published validation studies for these simulators. All three have publications establishing face, content, construct, and concurrent validation. There is only one published study on the predictive validity of the DVSS (Hung, 2012). Recent presentations explore the validity of the RoSS curriculum (Stegemann, 2013) and the RoSS' HoST procedural modules (Ahmed, 2013).

Table 7. Validation of robotic surgical simulators

Validation	DVSS	dV-Trainer	RoSS
Face	Hung 2011 Kelly 2012 Liss 2012	Lendvay 2008 Kenney 2009 Sethi 2009 Perrenot 2011 Korets, 2011 Lee 2012	Seixas-Mikelus 2010 Stegemann, 2012
Content	Hung 2011 Kelly 2012 Liss 2012	Kenney 2009 Sethi 2009 Perrenot 2011 Lee 2012	Seixas-Mikelus 2010 Colaco, 2012
Construct	Hung 2011 Kelly 2012 Liss 2012 Finnegan 2012	Kenney 2009 Korets, 2011 Perrenot 2011 Lee 2012	Raza, 2013
Concurrent	Hung 2012	Lerner 2010 Perrenot 2011 Korets 2011 Lee 2012	Chowriappa, 2013
Predictive	Hung 2012		

Section 6:
Conclusion

Simulators play an important role in providing training experience and a platform for evaluation of novices who are trying to master complex skills in many fields. When a task is simple, consequences for failure are minimal, and equipment is inexpensive, there is little motivation for creating a dedicated simulation device. However, when the task to be mastered is complex, there is a need for a device that can objectively measure the performance of the trainee and provide feedback that leads to improved performance. When the consequences of a mistake are lethal, there is a need for a safe environment in which to develop expertise without threatening the wellbeing of others. When equipment or disposables are expensive to use, there is a need for a tool that can provide at least entry-level familiarization and skill development without undue financial demands. All three of these conditions are characteristic of the process for learning robotic surgery. So it is not surprising that market forces have led to the creation of multiple simulators of the robotic system and the skills to use it.

The three simulators which are described in this book offer a different value proposition to potential purchasers and to novice learners. The da Vinci Skills Simulator, dV-Trainer, an RoSS are complex systems which are significantly less costly than the actual da Vinci robotic surgical system and can be operated at a fraction of the cost of the instruments required for this robot. The intent of this book is to present the characteristics of each system to enable intelligent and informed purchasing and usage decisions.

References

McDougall EM. , Validation of surgical simulators. *J Endourol.* 2007 Mar; 21(3):244-7.

da Vinci Skill Simulator

Skills Simulator for the da Vinci Si Surgical System, (Users Manual), Intuitive Surgical Inc., 2012.

Finnegan KT, Meraney AM, Staff I, da Vinci Skills Simulator construct validation study: correlation of prior robotic experience with overall score and time score simulator performance. *Urology.* 2012 Aug;80(2):330-5. doi: 10.1016/j.urology.2012.02.059. Epub 2012 Jun 15.

Hung AJ, Patil MB, Zehnder P, Concurrent and predictive validation of a novel robotic surgery simulator: a prospective, randomized study. *J Urol.* 2012 Feb;187(2):630-7.

Hung AJ, Zehnder P, Patil MB, Face, content and construct validity of a novel robotic surgery simulator. *J Urol.* 2011 Sep;186(3):1019-24.

Kelly DC, Margules AC, Kundavaram CR, Face, content, and construct validation of the da Vinci Skills Simulator. *Urology.* 2012 May;79(5):1068-72.

Liss MA, Abdelshehid C, Quach S, Validation, Correlation, and Comparison of the da Vinci Trainer(™) and the da Vinci Surgical Skills Simulator(™) Using the Mimic(™) Software for Urologic Robotic Surgical Education. *J Endourol.* 2012 Oct 2.

Sethi AS, Peine WJ, Mohammadi Y, Validation of a novel virtual reality robotic simulator. *J Endourol.* 2009 Mar;23(3):503-8.

dV-Trainer

dV-Trainer Robotic Simulator Users Manual, Mimic Technologies, Inc., 2012.

Kenney P, Wszolek M, Gould J, Libertino J, Moinzadeh A, "Face, Content, and Construct Validity of dV-Trainer, a Novel Virtual Reality Simulator for Robotic Surgery", *Journal of Urology*, Volume 73, Issue 6, June 2009.

Kim S, Cho J, "Validation Study of a 3D Virtual Robot Simulator as a Robot Surgery Training System", *Journal of Korean Colorectal Surgery*, April 2011.

Korets R, Graversen JA, Mues A, Gupta M, Landman J, Badani KK. Face and construct validity assessment of 2nd generation robotic surgery simulator. *J Urol* 2011; 185 (Suppl.): e488.

Korets R, Mues AC, Graversen JA, Gupta M, Benson MC, Cooper KL, Landman J, Badani KK, "Validating the Use of the Mimic dV-Trainer for Robotic Surgery Skill Acquisition Among Urology Residents", *Urology*, October 2011.

Lee JY, Mucksavage P, Kerbl DC Validation study of a virtual reality robotic simulator--role as an assessment tool? *J Urol.* 2012 Mar;187(3):998-1002. Epub 2012 Jan 20.

Lendvay TS, Casale P, Sweet R, VR robotic surgery: randomized blinded study of the dV-Trainer robotic simulator. *Stud Health Technol Inform.* 2008;132:242-4.

Lendvay, P. Casale, R. Sweet, C. Peters. Initial validation of a virtual-reality robotic simulator, *Journal of Robotic Surgery*, Volume 2, Number 3, September 2008.

Lerner M, Ayalew M, Peine W, Sundaram C,"Does Training on a Virtual Reality Robotic Simulator Improve Performance on the da Vinci® Surgical System?", *Journal of Endourology*, Volume 24, Number 3, March 2010.

Perrenot C, Perez M, Tran N, The virtual reality simulator dV-Trainer(®) is a valid assessment tool for robotic surgical skills. *Surg Endosc.* 2012 Sep;26(9):2587-93. doi: 10.1007/s00464-012-2237-0. Epub 2012 Apr 5.

Sethi AS, Peine WJ, Mohammadi Y, Validation of a novel virtual reality robotic simulator. *J Endourol.* 2009 Mar;23(3):503-8.

RoSS

Robotic Surgery Simulator Users Manual: For Models S and Si, Simulated Surgical Systems LLC, 2012.

Ahmed K, Chowriappa A, Din R, Field E, Raza SJ, Fazili A, Samarasekera D, Kaouk J, Eichel L, Joseph J, Ghazi A, Mohler J, Peabody J, Eun D, Shi Y, Wilding G, Kesavadas T, Guru KA, "A Multi-institutional Randomized Controlled Trial of an Augmented-Reality based technical skill acquisition module for Robot-assisted Urethro-vesical Anastomosis", Podium presentation, AUA Annual Congress, San Diego, May 4- 9, 2013.

Berry E, "Robotic Surgical Simulator advances training criteria for today's surgeons" Briefings on Credentialing May 1, 2010 (Vol. 19, Issue 5).

Chowriappa A, Raza SJ, Stegemann A, Ahmed K, Shi Y, Wilding G, Kaouk J, Peabody JO, Menon M, Kesavadas T, Guru KA, "Development & Validation of a Composite Grading & Scoring System for Robot-assisted Surgical Training—The Robotic Skills Assessment Scale", Podium presentation, AUA Annual Congress, San Diego, May 4- 9, 2013.

Colaco M, Balica A, Su D, Initial experiences with RoSS surgical simulator in residency training: a validity and model analysis, *J Robotic Surg*, DOI 10.1007/s11701-012-0376-x.

Guru K, Baheti A, Kesavadas T, Kumar A, Srimathveeravalli G, and Butt Z "In-Vivo Videos Enhance Cognitive Skills for da Vinci® Surgical System", *Journal of Urology* 181:4 Supplement, 2009.

Kesavadas T , Kumar A, Srimathveeravalli G, Karimpuzha S, Baheti A, Chandrasekhar R, Wilding G, Butt Z and Guru K "Efficacy of Robotic Surgery Simulator (RoSS) for the daVinci® Surgical System", *Journal of Urology* 181:4 Supplement, 2009.

Kesavadas T, Stegemann A, Sathyaseelan, G, Chowriappa A, Srimathveeravalli G, Seixas-Mikelus S, Chandrasekhar R, Wilding G, and Guru K. "Validation of Robotic Surgery Simulator (RoSS)", *Stud Health Technol Inform.* 2011;163:274-6.

Kumar A, Seshadri S, Baheti A, Srimathveeravalli G, Butt Z, Kuvshinoff B, Mohler J, Kesavadas T and Guru K "Virtual Reality Surgical Trainer for Robotic Urological Procedures" *Journal of Urology* 179:4:Supplement 1, 2008.

Raza SJ, Chowriappa A, Stegemann A, Ahmed K, Shi Y, Wilding G, Kaouk J, Peabody J, Menon M, Kesavadas T, Guru KA, "Construct Validation of the Fundamental Skills of Robotic Surgery (FSRS) Curriculum", Podium presentation, AUA Annual Congress, San Diego, May 4- 9, 2013.

Seixas-Mikelus S, Adal A, Srimathveeravalli G, Kesavadas T, Baheti A, Chandrashekar R, Wilding G and Guru K "Can Image Based Virtual Reality Help Teach Anatomy?" *Journal of Endourology*, Vol 24 (4), April 2010.

Seixas-Mikelus SA, Kesavadas T, Srimathveeravalli G, Face validation of a novel robotic surgical simulator. *Urology.* 2010 Aug;76(2):357-60. Epub 2010 Mar 17.

Seixas-Mikelus SA, Stegemann AP, Kesavadas T, Content validation of a novel robotic surgical simulator. *BJU Int.* 2011 Apr;107(7):1130-5.

Stegemann A, Kesavadas T, Rehman S, Sharif M, Rao M, duPont N, Shi Y, Wilding G, Hassett J, and Guru K, "Development, Implementation, and Validation of a Simulation-Based Curriculum for Robot-Assisted Surgery", *Urology* 2013 Apr;81(4):767-74.

Stegemann AP, Kesavadas T, Rehman S, Sharif M, Rao A, DuPont N, Shi Y, Wilding,G, Hassett J, and Guru K, "Development, Implementation and Validation of a Simulation-Based Curriculum for Robot-Assisted Surgery" Presented at the AUA poster session, May 19-23, 2012 Atlanta, GA.

Su D, and Barone J, "Initial Experience with the ROSS Robotic Simulator in Residency Training" moderated poster, AUA 2011.

Zorn K, and Gautam G, "Training, Credentialing, and Hospital Privileging for Robotic Urological Surgery", *Robotics in Genitourinary Surgery 2011*, Part 2, PP 169-181.

www.ingramcontent.com/pod-product-compliance
Lightning Source LLC
LaVergne TN
LVHW042351060326
832902LV00006B/536